# About me!

Greetings! I'm KS Kamboh, a seasoned doctor with a penchant for helping people navigate the complex landscape of their health. With my stethoscope as a trusted sidekick, I've embarked on a medical journey that's taken me from the bustling clinics of Pakistan to the rolling green hills of Ireland and now to the heart of the NHS in the UK.

But beyond the titles and the degrees, what truly drives me is the desire to make a difference in the lives of individuals like you. You see, I've had the privilege of working with countless patients, each with their unique set of health challenges. It's these interactions that have shaped my perspective and motivated me to share my knowledge with the world.

My goal has always been to demystify the world of medicine, to bridge the gap between healthcare professionals and the individuals seeking answers and support. So, join me on this journey. Let's explore the intriguing realm of health together, where I promise to be your trusted companion, helping you make informed decisions about your well-being and offering a friendly hand in the often bewildering maze of healthcare. So, welcome to my world. It's a pleasure to meet you!

# About This Book!

In this book, I wear many hats – that of a seasoned medical professional, a compassionate caregiver, and someone who's been personally touched by the challenges of COPD. What sets this book apart is that it's not just a compilation of dry facts and figures. No, it's a labor of love, a treasure trove of insights drawn from my experiences and those of my own family.

COPD (Chronic Obstructive Pulmonary Disease) is a complex condition, and in these pages, I've made it my mission to unravel its intricacies in a way that's easy to understand. I've been there, in the shoes of a doctor explaining a diagnosis to a patient, and as a son supporting his father through the ups and downs of COPD. That unique perspective, I believe, allows me to address the problems and questions that truly matter.

From understanding the causes of COPD to demystifying the diagnostic process, I've got you covered. But it doesn't stop there. This book delves deep into the intricacies of managing COPD, offering insights on everything from treatment options and post-management plans to the emotional support that's often needed along this journey.

We'll talk about diet, exercise, and lifestyle adjustments that can make a world of difference. And through it all, you'll find my friendly, empathetic voice, guiding you every step of the way.

So, consider this book your trusty companion on your COPD journey. Whether you're a patient, a caregiver, or just someone curious about this condition, I'm here to provide the answers and support you need. It's not just a book; it's a helping hand, a source of comfort, and a testament to the power of knowledge and understanding. Welcome to this journey – I'm excited to share it with you.

# Table of Contents

"COPD may slow me down, but it will never stop me from living my life to the fullest."

Chapter 1:

# Understanding COPD

## (Chronic Obstructive Pulmonary Disease)

## What is COPD, and Why Does It Happen?

Meet Sarah, a retired teacher with a love for gardening. She spent her days tending to her beautiful flowers and enjoying the peacefulness of her garden. However, over time, she noticed that something was amiss. She struggled to catch her breath, even on her way to the garden gate. This concerned her, so she decided to learn more about what was happening. So she visits her GP. After assessment, GP tells her she might have COPD & needs more tests to confirm. COPD? But what's that?

Well, COPD sounds complicated, but let's break it down with a story:

Once upon a time, in a faraway land called LungsVille, there lived a brave knight named Sir Breaths-a-Lot. His job was to keep the air flowing freely into and out of the two magical balloons inside his chest, which he called "lungs." But as the years passed, a sneaky dragon named Mr. Smoke arrived in LungsVille. Mr. Smoke blew his fiery breath into Sir Breaths-a-Lot's lungs, making them weaker and less stretchy. Sir Breaths-a-Lot found it harder to breathe, just like Sarah did.
So, COPD is like a dragon that weakens the magical balloons in your chest, making it tough to breathe.

## What are Causes of COPD?

Now, you might wonder how this dragon got into LungsVille in the first place. Well, let's consider another story:

Imagine a cozy cabin deep in the forest, where Grandma Cook, a wise old woman, loved to prepare delicious meals. She often used firewood to cook, but the smoke from the wood wasn't just yummy smells; it was also filled with tiny, invisible villains that hurt the lungs. Spending years in Grandma Cook's cabin, even if you weren't a fire-breathing dragon like Mr. Smoke, could make your lungs weak, just like **smoking** does. Remember, even if you've never smoked, other things like dusty workplaces, pollution, and wood smoke can let these invisible villains into your lungs.

## What are different Types of COPD?

Now, let's dive into the world of COPD types. Yes, there's not just one, but a whole ensemble of them. Think of it as meeting the various characters in a story. Each type has its unique features and quirks, and we'll make it engaging and even a little funny along the way. So, let's get to know our COPD cast!

## 1.Chronic Bronchitis

Our first character is Chronic Bronchitis, or as we like to call it, "**The Cough King**." This type of COPD is all about a chronic, persistent cough and excessive mucus production. It's like a never-ending symphony of coughs, hacking, and throat clearing. If you're into humor, you might say it's your body's way of auditioning for the next great coughing contest. Chronic bronchitis is often accompanied by shortness of breath and fatigue.

## 2. Emphysema

Next up is Emphysema, also known as "The Lung Elastinator." It's like the neighborhood trampoline gone wrong – your lung tissues lose their elasticity, and it becomes harder for them to bounce back. This makes it difficult for air to flow in and out, causing that notorious shortness of breath, also known as the "panting protagonist." Emphysema often leads to barrel chest, which is like the lung's way of making a fashion statement.

## 3. Overlapping COPD

Now, let's talk about the ultimate crossover episode – Overlapping COPD. It's like the superhero team-up movie of lung diseases. In this scenario, individuals can have both chronic bronchitis and emphysema simultaneously. It's like battling two foes at once, making symptoms more challenging and sometimes requiring a double strategy for treatment.

## 4. Asthma-COPD Overlap

Imagine a cop and a detective teaming up to solve a case; that's what happens when COPD and asthma join forces. This is known as the Asthma-COPD Overlap, or ACOS for short. It's like having two troublemakers in your airways. ACOS combines the airway obstruction seen in COPD with the wheezing and inflammation seen in asthma. It's like a turbulent partnership between partners in crime.

## 5. Bronchiectasis

Meet Bronchiectasis, or as we like to call it, "The Dilation Dynamo." It's like your airways have decided to expand and stay that way. This can lead to the accumulation of mucus and a constant cycle of infections. Bronchiectasis is like the curious explorer of the COPD world, making you prone to persistent cough and infections.

And there you have it, the fabulous cast of COPD characters! Just like in a play or movie, each type of COPD has its unique role and characteristics. Whether it's the coughing king, the lung elastinator, the crossover episode, the dynamic duo, or the dilation dynamo, understanding these types can help you and your healthcare team tailor your management plan.

## What are Stages and Severity of COPD?

COPD comes in different stages, like the colors of a traffic light. Imagine you're driving down the road, and your breath is your car:

- **Stage 1 (Mild - Green Light):** Think of this as cruising along with a green light. You might hit a little traffic, but it's not too bad. Just like a small traffic jam doesn't stop you completely, mild COPD only makes breathing a bit tricky.
- **Stage 2 (Moderate - Yellow Light):** Now, picture a yellow light. It's a warning, like when you see a school bus stopping. Breathing is getting harder, especially when you do activities. You're slowing down.
- **Stage 3 (Severe - Red Light):** Imagine a big, red traffic light. It's a full stop. Breathing is really tough, and simple things like climbing stairs or going for a walk feel like running a marathon.
- **Stage 4 (Very Severe - Emergency - Stop!):** Here, it's not just a red light; it's a giant stop sign. Breathing is extremely difficult, and you might even need help from a machine to get enough air, just like when there's a roadblock.

## What are Common Symptoms and Warning Signs?

The signs of COPD are like red flags trying to get your attention:

- **Chronic Cough:** Imagine having a friend who coughs all the time, not because they're sick, but because something is bothering their lungs. It's a bit like having a tickly feather stuck in your throat that won't go away.

- **Shortness of Breath:** Think about climbing a hill and feeling out of breath. Now, imagine feeling like that even when you're doing simple things like folding laundry or setting the table for dinner.

- **Wheezing:** Remember blowing up a balloon and the funny noise it makes? Wheezing is like that sound but coming from your chest when you breathe, just like a squeaky toy that needs some oil.

- **Chest Tightness:** Picture someone giving you a big hug that's too tight. That's how some people describe the feeling in their chest, like a jacket that's a size too small.

- **Respiratory Infections:** Sometimes, your lungs can get infected easily. It's like having a door that's not quite closed, letting in troublemakers. It's a bit like a house with a broken window where pests can enter.

- **Fatigue:** Imagine trying to carry a heavy backpack all day long. Your shoulders get tired, and your body feels worn out. That's how some people feel because their lungs are working extra hard.

- **Unintended Weight Loss:** If you're not as interested in food because you're too tired or breathless, you might lose weight without meaning to, like an explorer who forgets to pack snacks for the journey.

- **Frequent Clearing of Throat**: You might have the constant urge to clear your throat, as mucus and irritation can build up in the airways.

- **Decreased Exercise Tolerance**: You may notice that you can't engage in physical activities for as long as you used to, and you might need more rest during exercise.

- **Difficulty Doing Daily Activities**: Simple activities such as walking, climbing stairs, or carrying groceries can become increasingly challenging due to shortness of breath and fatigue.

- **Blueness of Lips or Fingernails (Cyanosis)**: In severe cases of COPD, when the blood oxygen levels drop significantly, the skin, lips, or fingertips may turn bluish due to insufficient oxygen.

Just like Sarah, if you notice any of these signs in yourself or a loved one, it's important to see a doctor. They can help you figure out what's going on and what steps to take next. Your journey may have its own unique story, but understanding COPD can help you navigate it more successfully.

"You can and will be able to make a significant difference in the quality of your life if you make the commitment to take an active role in managing your disease". – Teri Allen

Chapter 2:

# Unmasking the Culprits: What's Behind COPD?

In this chapter, we're going to unveil the mysterious causes behind COPD – Chronic Obstructive Pulmonary Disease. Think of it as unmasking the villains of the story, but don't worry; we'll keep it light and maybe even a little funny. After all, laughter is the best medicine, and we could all use a good laugh!

So, grab your detective hats, and let's embark on this journey to uncover the secrets that lead to COPD. Spoiler alert: the culprits might be right under your nose, or should I say, in your lungs!

## 1. The Smoking Gun

Alright, let's address the elephant in the room (or should I say the cloud of smoke?). The most notorious culprit in the development of COPD is smoking. It's like the Sherlock Holmes of lung diseases. Smoking, whether it's cigarettes, cigars, or even a pipe, or even vape, is like inviting trouble right into your lungs.

You see, the chemicals and toxins in tobacco smoke wage an all-out war on your lungs. They irritate the airways, inflame the lung tissues, and lead to the production of mucus. Over time, this relentless assault can narrow your airways and make it harder to breathe. So, if you're looking for a good laugh, do yourself a favor – quit smoking!

## 2. The Second hand Bandit

Now, let's talk about secondhand smoke. It's like a sneak attack from the shadows. Even if you're not the one puffing away, being around smokers can expose you to harmful chemicals. It's like being an innocent bystander in a crime movie – you didn't do anything wrong, but you're caught in the crossfire.

Exposure to secondhand smoke can lead to the same lung troubles as smoking. So, be a detective in your own life and avoid smoky situations. It's a win-win – you'll protect your lungs and your friends' lungs at the same time.

## 3. Occupational Hazards

Sometimes, your workplace can be a breeding ground for COPD culprits. You might be dealing with dust, fumes, or other airborne nasties. Jobs like mining, construction, and textile work can be particularly risky. These occupational hazards are like cunning villains, lurking in the background.

Inhaling these occupational hazards day in and day out can lead to lung irritation and inflammation. It's like a long, slow burn, and eventually, it can build up to COPD. So, if your job has you mingling with lung irritants, make sure you take protective measures and use appropriate safety equipment.

## 4. Alpha-1 Antitrypsin (Enzyme) Deficiency

Now, for the more mysterious culprit – Alpha-1 Antitrypsin Deficiency. It's like the hidden traitor within your own body. You see, our bodies have a natural defense system to protect our lungs. Alpha-1 Antitrypsin is one of the good guys, and its job is to keep an eye on an enzyme called elastase, which can break down lung tissue.

But sometimes, due to genetics, the body doesn't produce enough of this protective protein. It's like having a bouncer at the club who's too busy chatting up the DJ to keep troublemakers out. Without enough Alpha-1 Antitrypsin, your lungs are more vulnerable to damage, leading to COPD.

## 5. Genetics, The Silent Partner

It's not always about lifestyle or occupational exposure. Genetics can play a role too, and it's like having a silent partner in the crime. If you have a family history of COPD, you might be at higher risk. It's like inheriting a not-so-great trait from your ancestors.

Sometimes, genes can predispose you to develop COPD, even without significant exposure to smoke or other lung irritants. But don't worry, knowing your family history can help you stay one step ahead and be proactive about your lung health.


## 5. Respiratory Infections

Now, let's talk about the opportunistic villains – respiratory infections. If you've had your fair share of lung infections, like pneumonia or frequent bronchitis, it can contribute to the development of COPD. It's like inviting trouble to your doorstep.

These infections can damage your airways and lung tissues, leaving scars behind. Over time, this can make your airways narrower and more obstructed, making breathing a real challenge.

And there you have it, dear readers – the culprits behind COPD. It's like solving a complex mystery, but now you're equipped with the knowledge to protect yourself and your loved ones. Whether it's quitting smoking, avoiding secondhand smoke, being cautious at work, or understanding your genetic risks, you can be your own lung health detective.

Remember, laughter might be a great medicine, but taking care of your lungs is the best prescription. So, let's keep those lungs happy and healthy as we continue our journey through the world of COPD.

"You can find your best life with COPD — a life with health, happiness, and hope." – Jane Martin

Chapter 3:

# The Great COPD Detective: Unmasking the Diagnosis

In this chapter, we're going to embark on an investigative journey into the world of COPD diagnosis. Think of it as donning your detective hat and magnifying glass. We'll explore the tools and tricks used to confirm COPD in its early and later stages, helping you understand the need and reasons for different tests which are necessary at certain times throughout your journey.

## Step 1: Medical History – The Initial Clues

Our detective story begins with the most straightforward step: your medical history. Think of it as the first page of a mystery novel, where you share your health story. Your healthcare provider will ask about your symptoms, risk factors like smoking history, and any family history of lung disease. It's like revealing the initial clues that lead us to the mystery's heart.

## Step 2: Physical Examination – The Visual Inspection

Next up is the physical examination, our version of Sherlock Holmes' keen observation. Your healthcare provider will listen to your chest, looking for telltale signs like wheezing or unusual breathing sounds. They might also check your fingers for "clubbing," which can be a hint that something's amiss. It's like scanning the crime scene for evidence.

## Step 3: Spirometry – The COPD Interrogation

Now, it's time to bring in the heavy artillery – spirometry. Spiro-what? It's like strapping a lie detector on your lungs. You take a deep breath and then exhale forcefully into a machine, which measures your lung capacity and how fast you can blow out the air. It's one of the most important tools for diagnosing COPD, helping to confirm whether you have airflow obstruction.

## Step 4: Pulmonary Function Tests – The Stress Test

Pulmonary function tests (PFTs) are like the stress test of our investigation. They give more detailed information about your lung function. Imagine this as your lungs' time in the spotlight, showing off their capabilities. PFTs include various measurements to assess how well your lungs are functioning, such as lung volumes, diffusion capacity, and the response to bronchodilators.

## Step 5: Chest X-ray – The Visual Evidence

A chest X-ray is like the surveillance footage in our investigation. It provides a visual check of your lungs and surrounding structures. While it might not directly confirm COPD, it can rule out other conditions or show signs of complications, like pneumonia or lung cancer. It's an essential piece of the puzzle.

## Step 6: CT Scan – The Deep Dive

In some cases, a CT scan is needed. Think of it as our deep-dive detective tool, like a magnifying glass for your insides. It provides a more detailed look at your lungs and can help spot emphysema or other lung conditions that might be masquerading as COPD.

## Blood Tests – The Clue Hunt

Blood tests are like hunting for clues in the mystery. They can help identify or rule out other conditions that might be affecting your lungs. For example, they can measure your oxygen and carbon dioxide levels, check for signs of infection, or assess whether you have alpha-1 antitrypsin deficiency.

## Arterial Blood Gas – The Bloodhound

Arterial blood gas (ABG) tests are like our trusty bloodhound sniffing out leads. They measure the levels of oxygen and carbon dioxide in your blood. This test helps determine how well your lungs are exchanging gases, which can be especially helpful if you have severe COPD or an sudden attack of COPD.

## Bronchoscopy – The Detective's Specialized Tool

Bronchoscopy is like our detective's secret weapon. It's an invasive procedure where a thin, flexible tube with a camera is inserted into your airways to get a closer look. This can help rule out other conditions and might be used if your diagnosis is still unclear.

## Final Confirmation – The Smoking Gun

Once all the pieces are in place, your healthcare provider will put it all together. It's like the dramatic reveal in a classic detective novel. If you have a history of smoking, persistent symptoms, abnormal spirometry results, and other supporting evidence, the diagnosis of COPD becomes clearer.

And there you have it, dear readers – the complete guide to the diagnosis of COPD. It's like piecing together a puzzle, with each step providing essential clues to confirm the diagnosis. Whether it's the initial medical history, physical examination, spirometry, pulmonary function tests, imaging, blood tests, or even the specialized tools like bronchoscopy, each plays a unique role in our great COPD detective story. Now depending on specific situations of each person, tests required may vary. You don't need to go through all those tests to confirm the diagnosis of COPD. Long smoking history and persistent signs and symptoms usually give a clue which is later confirmed with spirometry and Lung function tests. Medications are only needed if you become symptomatic.

Remember, early detection is crucial, as it allows for better management and improved quality of life. So, put on your detective hat and work closely with your healthcare team to unmask the COPD culprit.

"It's important to educate yourself now versus later. Knowledge is power, and having all the knowledge at the start will make the rest of the journey that much easier to deal with."

# Chapter 4

# The COPD Odyssey: Navigating the Seas of Management

Let's now  explore the various strategies and tools you can use to keep your COPD ship afloat. So, hoist the anchor, set the sails, and let's embark on this journey to manage COPD from the early stages to the final showdown!

## Early Stages - The Smokescreen of Smoking Cessation

Let's start where it all begins - the early stages. If you're a smoker, the first and funniest step is to quit smoking. Think of it as ditching the villain in your life, the evil twin of COPD. It's not just about willpower; you can use nicotine replacement therapies or medications to help. And you know what they say, quitting smoking is like breaking up with a really bad ex – you'll feel much better afterward!

## Lung-Boosting Lifestyle Changes

As you navigate these early waters, lifestyle changes become your trusty first mate. Exercise is your sword, and a healthy diet is your shield. It's like preparing for a medieval battle; you need to stay strong and resilient. Regular physical activity can improve your lung function and stamina, while a balanced diet helps fuel your body's defenses. Think of it as building a moat around your lung castle.

## Medications - Your COPD Arsenal

Now, let's talk about the real firepower - medications. In the early stages, you might use bronchodilators, like albuterol, to help open up your airways. It's like having a mini jet engine for your lungs, providing quick relief when you need it.

In more advanced stages, you may meet your long-term partners, the inhaled corticosteroids and long-acting bronchodilators. They're like the Bonnie and Clyde of COPD management, working together to reduce inflammation and keep your airways open. These medications can be delivered through inhalers, nebulizers, or even pills.

## Pulmonary Rehabilitation – Your COPD Boot Camp

Think of pulmonary rehabilitation as your COPD boot camp – it's where you whip those lungs into shape. You'll work with a team of experts who will help you with exercises, breathing techniques, and nutritional advice. It's like a superhero training montage from a movie, but you're the hero!

## Oxygen Therapy – The Lifesaver Balloon

In more advanced stages of COPD, you might need oxygen therapy. Picture it like carrying around a helium balloon that never floats away. It provides that precious oxygen your body craves, helping you breathe easier. It's like having your personal air supply, making you feel like an astronaut on a spacewalk.

## Advanced Treatments – The Magic Wands

When the seas get stormy, you have advanced treatments like theophylline, which is like a magic wand that opens your airways further. Or there's roflumilast, which can help reduce lung inflammation. It's like having a secret weapon against COPD.

## Surgical Options – The Ship Repair Crew

In the most severe cases, you may need surgical interventions. Procedures like lung volume reduction surgery or even a lung transplant can be considered. It's like sending in the ship repair crew to patch up your vessel. These are the big guns, used when other treatments don't cut it.

## End-of-Life Care – Facing the Kraken

Lastly, let's talk about end-of-life care. It's like facing the Kraken – the final battle. When the time comes, palliative care and hospice care can provide comfort and support. It's not giving up; it's ensuring you have the best quality of life possible in the face of the most challenging enemy.

And there you have it, the epic journey of COPD management. From quitting smoking to lung-boosting lifestyle changes, medications, pulmonary rehabilitation, oxygen therapy, advanced treatments, surgical options, and end-of-life care, you've got a vast toolkit at your disposal.

COPD is like a turbulent adventure on the high seas, but with the right strategies, you can navigate the waters and make it through. Remember, you're the captain of this ship, and the winds of management are at your command. So, keep sailing forward, and keep your morale high.

*Next few Chapters contain further details of each section in COPD Management

"You are more than your lung disease" – John Landry

Chapter 5:

# Medications and Treatment – Breathing Easier

Imagine you have a magical tool chest, and inside, there are different tools to help you feel better and breathe more comfortably. In the world of COPD, these tools are like medications. Let's open the chest and see what's inside:

- **Bronchodilators (Airway Openers):** These are like keys that unlock the doors in your lungs to make breathing easier. Think of short-acting bronchodilators as quick keys you use when needed (like a spare key for your car), and long-acting bronchodilators as the master keys you use every day. Long acting ones are for long term to keep your airways open so that you don't have any problem breathing during the day. The short acting ones are for acute attacks, to give you instant relief.

- **Inhaled Corticosteroids (Lung Soothers):** These are like firefighters who calm the flames in your lungs and reduce the production of mucus. They work best when combined with bronchodilators for more severe COPD. Remember Sarah? On days when her COPD acts up, Sarah uses an inhaler with corticosteroids to help put out the "fire" in her lungs and breathe more freely.

- **Phosphodiesterase-4 Inhibitors (Peacekeepers):** Think of these as peacekeepers who maintain calm in your airways by controlling inflammation, especially when other treatments aren't enough. Sometimes, even with her other medications, Sarah's COPD flares up. So, her doctor prescribes a phosphodiesterase-4 inhibitor to maintain peace in her airways.

- **Antibiotics and Vaccines (Lung Guardians):** These are like guards protecting your lungs from invaders like bacteria and viruses, which can be especially important for people with COPD, who are more prone to infections. Every year, Sarah gets her flu shot and ensures she has her pneumonia vaccine to keep her lungs guarded against these invaders.

## Inhaler Techniques and Proper Use:

An inhaler is like a magic wand that can help you breathe more comfortably. Using it properly is essential. Here's how to do it:

- **Shake and Spray:** Give your inhaler a little shake, like you would a bottle of salad dressing. Stand up straight, take a deep breath, and exhale slowly. As you breathe in, put the inhaler to your lips, release the medicine, and continue to inhale slowly. Hold your breath for about 10 seconds, letting the medicine work its magic.

- **Spacer Magic:** Some inhalers come with a spacer, which makes it easier to get the medicine deep into your lungs. It's like having a helper for your magic wand. Attach the spacer to your inhaler, breathe in slowly, and let the spacer assist in getting the medicine where it's needed.

## The Role of Oxygen Therapy:

Oxygen therapy is like a boost of energy for your body when your lungs need extra help:

- **Portable Tanks:** These are like your personal oxygen supply. You can carry a portable tank with you, much like a water bottle, to have oxygen when you need it. They are usually required when disease is very severe & you're not able to retain enough oxygen in your body.

- **Concentrators:** At home, you might have an oxygen concentrator, which is like a mini-factory that turns regular air into oxygen-rich air. You can use a tube, like a straw, to breathe in this oxygen.

Like Sarah, finding the right combination of medications and treatment techniques can make a big difference in managing COPD. Your doctor is your guide, helping you discover which tools and techniques work best for your unique journey toward easier breathing and a more comfortable life.

"COPD is not a death sentence; it's a life sentence. It's a constant battle but one that is worth fighting."

Chapter 6:

# Smoking!
# "Quit or Not to Quit? That Is the Question"

Ladies and gentlemen, welcome to the grand theater of COPD, where the leading role is played by none other than the cunning villain - smoking. In this chapter, we're going to explore the importance of smoking cessation. Think of it as a Shakespearean tragedy where smoking takes center stage, and you're the hero deciding to quit or not to quit. We'll uncover the vital reasons for quitting and how it impacts every stage of COPD, from early to the very last act.

## Act 1: The Dangers of Smoking - "The Smoke Monster"

Let's start with Act 1 - The Dangers of Smoking. Smoking is like the smoke monster from a thriller – it's mysterious, dangerous, and capable of causing a lot of trouble. The fact is, smoking is the leading cause of COPD, and it doesn't stop there. It's also responsible for heart disease, cancer, and a host of other health issues which eventually contribute to making breathing even worse. But here's the kicker - quitting smoking at any stage is like defeating the smoke monster and reclaiming your life.

## Act 2: The Early Stages of COPD - "The Smokey Prelude"

Now, let's move to Act 2 - The Early Stages of COPD. It's like the smokey prelude to the main event. In the early stages, quitting smoking is your best buddy. Why? Because it helps slow down the progression of COPD. It's like hitting the brakes on a runaway train. Plus, you'll notice improvements in your symptoms and lung function, which is like getting your groove back.

## Act 3: The Intermediate Stages - "The Foggy Middle"

In Act 3, we're in the intermediate stages. It's like the foggy middle of a movie where things start to get intense. If you keep smoking, your COPD will likely worsen. You'll find yourself gasping for breath more often, and your quality of life will take a nosedive. But if you quit, you'll be like the action hero who saves the day, because quitting can help prevent further lung damage.

## Act 4: The Advanced Stages – "The Climactic Battle"

In Act 4, we've reached the advanced stages of COPD. It's like the climactic battle scene. If you keep smoking, your symptoms will become even more severe, and you'll need more medications and oxygen therapy to breathe. But if you quit, you'll be like the hero who faces the biggest challenge and prevails. Quitting can slow the progression of COPD, making your life more manageable.

## Act 5: End-of-Life Care – "The Final Act"

In Act 5, we've reached the final act, like end-of-life care. It's a somber moment, but it's also a moment of truth. Even if you're in the advanced stages, quitting smoking can still make a difference. It won't reverse the damage, but it can improve your quality of life and may even extend your time with loved ones. It's like making the most of your final scene.

## The Encore – "A Smoke-Free Life"

The grand finale, the encore, is the best part. A smoke-free life is like a standing ovation from the audience. You gain so much when you quit – better breathing, improved quality of life, and a chance to live healthier. Quitting smoking is the ultimate plot twist, turning the story from tragedy to triumph.

## To Quit or Not to Quit?

In the grand theater of life, quitting smoking is your best performance. It's the role of a lifetime, where you're the star. The importance of smoking cessation cannot be overstated. It's your ticket to a better, healthier, and longer life, no matter which act of COPD you find yourself in. So, to quit or not to quit? The answer is clear – quit and be the hero of your own story!

"COPD is not a sprint; it's a marathon. It requires patience, determination, and a strong will."

Chapter 7:

# Lifestyle Changes – A Breath of Fresh Air

Sarah's journey continues as she learns about the lifestyle changes that can make a big difference in managing her COPD. Let's join her in exploring these essential aspects of a healthier life.

## 1. Importance of Quitting Smoking (If Applicable):

Imagine you have a friend named Joe who loves playing with fire. One day, he starts a small fire, and even though it's fun at first, it quickly grows out of control. Now, Joe is stuck trying to put out the fire while it keeps getting bigger. Smoking is a bit like Joe's love for fire, but instead of playing, you're harming your lungs. Sarah used to smoke, but she realized it was like starting a fire in her own lungs. When she quit, she stopped adding fuel to that fire and gave her lungs a chance to heal.

Quitting smoking is like taking away the fuel that makes COPD worse. It's a challenge, but with the right support, you can do it, just like Sarah did.

## 2. Benefits of a Healthy Diet and Exercise:

Imagine your body is like a car. It needs good fuel (food) and regular maintenance (exercise) to run smoothly. Now, picture a car with a dirty engine and bad fuel; it sputters and doesn't go very far. But when you clean the engine and use high-quality fuel, it purrs like a kitten and takes you wherever you want.

- **A Healthy Diet:** Think of it as high-quality fuel for your body. Fresh fruits, vegetables, lean proteins, and whole grains are like the premium gasoline for your engine. They give you the energy you need to tackle your day. Sarah noticed that eating more fruits and vegetables made her feel more energetic. It was like putting the best fuel in her engine.

- **Exercise:** Consider it your regular maintenance. When you exercise, you're like a mechanic fine-tuning your engine. You don't need to run a marathon, but even a daily walk can help keep everything running smoothly. Sarah started taking short walks around her garden. It was like giving her engine regular check-ups to ensure everything was in good shape.

## 3. Breathing Techniques and Pulmonary Rehabilitation Programs:

Now, imagine you're a musician learning to play a new instrument, like a flute. At first, it's challenging, and you need to practice. But with the right guidance and exercises, you get better. Breathing techniques and pulmonary rehabilitation programs are a bit like music lessons for your lungs.

- **Breathing Techniques*:** These are simple exercises that help you use your lung capacity more effectively. They're like learning how to play the flute, starting with the basics and gradually getting better. Sarah practiced deep breathing exercises. It was like learning to play beautiful melodies with her lungs, making her breathe easier.

- **Pulmonary Rehabilitation Programs:** Think of these programs as your music school for better breathing. Just like a music teacher guides you in playing the flute, these programs provide you with expert guidance on managing your breathing and staying active. Sarah attended pulmonary rehabilitation, which was like her personal flute teacher helping her master the art of better breathing.

Remember, the journey to better lung health might have its challenges, but it's filled with opportunities to make your life more enjoyable and comfortable.

## *Breath Easy - The art of Breathing for COPD Patients:

Breathing is a bit like a comedy of errors. Most of us take it for granted, but when you have COPD, it can feel like a stand-up comedy show gone wrong. The simple act of breathing can become a challenge, leaving you gasping for air. That's where breathing exercises come in. They're like the comedy script for your lungs, teaching you how to breathe more efficiently and feel better.

### The Importance of Breathing Exercises

First things first, why do breathing exercises matter? Well, they're like your secret weapon in the battle against COPD. When you have COPD, your lung function isn't at its best. Breathing exercises can help you maximize what lung function you have left, making it easier to catch your breath, reduce symptoms, and improve your overall quality of life.

### Pursed Lip Breathing - The Lipstick Trick

Imagine pursed lip breathing as the lipstick trick of breathing exercises. Here's how it works: you take a breath in through your nose, and then exhale slowly through pursed lips, like you're blowing out a candle. It's like telling your lungs to take their time and savor the moment. Pursed lip breathing helps keep your airways open longer, making each breath more effective.

### Diaphragmatic Breathing - The Belly Laugh

Diaphragmatic breathing is like a good belly laugh – it's contagious, and it feels fantastic. This exercise focuses on your diaphragm, the main muscle used for breathing. To do it, place one hand on your chest and the other on your belly. Breathe in deeply through your nose, letting your belly rise like a balloon, and then exhale slowly through pursed lips. It's like teaching your diaphragm to do the heavy lifting for you.

## Huff Cough - The Gentle Reminder

The huff cough is like a gentle reminder to your lungs to clear out the gunk. It's simple but effective. Take a deep breath in, and then exhale with a series of three short, forceful exhales. It's like the polite way of telling mucus to hit the road. Huff cough helps move mucus from the smaller airways into the larger ones, making it easier to cough up.

## Controlled Coughing - The Grand Finale

Controlled coughing is like the grand finale of your breathing exercises. It's the showstopper when you need to clear mucus from your airways. Here's how it's done: Sit up straight, take a deep breath in through your nose, and then exhale slowly through pursed lips. After that, take a deep breath and give one good, strong cough. It's like the diva's high note, and it's excellent for moving mucus out of your lungs.

## Interval Training - The HIIT of Breathing

Interval training is like the HIIT (High-Intensity Interval Training) of breathing exercises. It's all about mixing things up to improve your lung capacity. For example, take a few deep breaths in, and then exhale slowly. Next, take quick, shallow breaths. It's like lung calisthenics, challenging your lung muscles and helping you breathe more efficiently.

## Relaxation Breathing - The Zen Master

Relaxation breathing is like becoming the Zen master of your breath. It's all about finding your inner peace and reducing anxiety, which can worsen COPD symptoms. To do it, sit or lie down comfortably, close your eyes, and take slow, deep breaths. Imagine inhaling calm and exhaling stress. It's like a mental spa day for your lungs.

Breathing exercises aren't just a one-time show; they're like the background music in your life. You can seamlessly blend them into your daily routine. Practice these exercises while watching your favorite TV show, waiting for your morning coffee to brew, or even during a leisurely stroll. The key is consistency; it's like practicing the piano until you become a maestro.

In the grand scheme of COPD management, breathing exercises are like the unsung heroes. They might not wear capes, but they have the power to improve your lung function, reduce symptoms, and enhance your quality of life. Think of it as the breathing revolution, where you take charge of your breath and make each one count.

"I may have COPD, but COPD does not have me."

Chapter 8:

# Managing Symptoms – Breathing Easy

In this chapter, we join Sarah as she continues her journey toward better managing her COPD symptoms. Let's explore some practical tips and strategies for dealing with shortness of breath, managing cough and mucus production, and recognizing and handling exacerbations or flare-ups.

## Dealing with Shortness of Breath:

Imagine your body is like a finely tuned car engine, but sometimes it struggles to get enough air. When you feel short of breath, it's like the engine is sputtering. You don't need to be a mechanic to help your body run smoothly. Here are some tips:

- **Pursed-Lip Breathing:** This technique is like putting the engine in low gear. Breathe in slowly through your nose for a count of two, and then exhale through pursed lips for a count of four. It helps to keep the airways open and can make breathing feel less strenuous. Sarah often uses pursed-lip breathing while gardening. It's like gently easing her engine into a lower gear, making it easier to keep going.

- **Practice Good Posture:** Imagine your body as a well-balanced car. Slumping or hunching over can put extra pressure on your lungs, making it harder to breathe. Sit or stand up straight to give your lungs more room. Sarah realized that when she stood tall, it was like her body's suspension system working better, allowing her to breathe more freely.

- **Control Anxiety:** Feeling anxious can make you breathe faster and shallower, worsening shortness of breath. Techniques like deep breathing and relaxation exercises can help you stay calm. Sarah found that when she practiced deep breathing exercises during stressful moments, it was like calming her racing engine and helping it run more smoothly.

## Strategies for Managing Cough and Mucus Production:

Now, imagine that mucus in your airways is like leaves clogging a drain. Clearing it out is like having a good maintenance routine. Here are some strategies to help manage cough and mucus:

- **Stay Hydrated:** Think of water as the solution to thinning mucus. Like pouring warm water down a clogged drain to clear it, drinking enough fluids helps keep mucus less sticky and easier to clear. Sarah keeps a bottle of water handy in her garden, sipping it frequently. It's like using a hose to keep the drains clear.

- **Use a Humidifier:** A humidifier adds moisture to the air, like a gentle rain clearing the way. It can help thin mucus, making it easier to cough up. Sarah places a humidifier in her bedroom. It's like having a little cloud over her garden, making the air easier to breathe.

- **Control Allergens:** Like keeping your house clean to prevent dust and dirt from clogging your engine, reducing exposure to allergens can help control mucus production. Use air purifiers and keep your home free from irritants like pet dander and smoke. Sarah noticed that reducing allergens in her home was like keeping the engine room clean and well-maintained, making her breathing easier.

## Recognizing and Handling Exacerbations or Flare-Ups:

Imagine your body as a car engine with a warning light. When that light comes on, it's like a flare-up or exacerbation in COPD. Knowing how to handle it is like a good mechanic diagnosing and fixing the problem. Here's how to recognize and manage flare-ups:

- **Recognize Early Warning Signs:** Just like the car's warning light, your body gives you clues. Watch out for increased shortness of breath, worsening cough, or changes in the color or thickness of mucus.

- **Follow an Action Plan:** Like a mechanic using a manual to fix the engine, work with your healthcare provider to create a COPD action plan. This plan outlines what to do when symptoms worsen, including which medications to use and when to seek medical help.

- **Stay Prepared:** Keep your medications and important documents (like your action plan and medical records) handy. It's like having a well-equipped toolbox in case you need to fix something in the car engine.

- **Seek Medical Help Promptly:** When the warning light in your car stays on, it's time to see the mechanic. Similarly, when your COPD symptoms worsen and don't improve with your action plan, it's essential to contact your healthcare provider. They can assess your condition and adjust your treatment as needed.

By following these tips for shortness of breath, strategies for managing cough and mucus, and recognizing and handling exacerbations, you can be like a skilled mechanic, keeping your body's engine running smoothly and avoiding major breakdowns. Just like Sarah, you can navigate the twists and turns of living with COPD, making the journey more manageable and comfortable.

"Fear less, hope more; eat less, chew more;
whine less, breathe more; talk less, say more;
hate less, love more; and all good things are
yours."

Chapter 9:

# Home Environment – Crafting Your COPD friendly Heaven

In this chapter, we'll embark on a journey to create a home environment that's as comforting as your favorite pair of slippers. With COPD in the passenger seat, we're going to explore the art of making your home a place where you can breathe easy, improve your indoor air quality, and ensure you've got your safety belt on with essential emergency plans.

## Creating a COPD-Friendly Home Environment

Imagine your home as your castle, your sanctuary, and with a bit of creative flair, we'll turn it into a COPD-friendly oasis:

- **Clear the Clutter:** Just as a messy car can make your road trip a headache, a cluttered home can make breathing a chore. Keep your living spaces tidy and obstacle-free. This isn't just cleaning; it's decluttering for your lungs!

- **Opt for Easy-to-Clean Surfaces:** Carpets and heavy curtains are like magnets for dust and allergens, making your home air feel like a dust storm. Swap them for smooth, easy-to-clean surfaces like hardwood floors and blinds. It's like rolling out a red carpet for your breath.

- **Create a Restful Bedroom:** Your bedroom is your zen den, your ticket to dreamland. Invest in a comfy mattress, hypoallergenic bedding, and keep the room well-ventilated. A good night's sleep is like a pit stop for your energy levels.

- **Consider a Home Air Purifier:** Think of an air purifier as your home's personal lung spa. It filters out particles and allergens, making your indoor air feel like a breath of fresh air. Breathe in, breathe out, and relax.

## Improving Indoor Air Quality and Reducing Triggers

Let's talk about indoor air quality - it's like the aroma of a brand new car, but better:

- **Ventilate Your Home:** Fresh air is like a breath of mountain air on a road trip. Use exhaust fans in the kitchen and bathroom, and open windows to invite clean outdoor air inside. It's your home's way of saying "welcome!"

- **Keep Humidity in Check:** Too much moisture is like inviting mold and dust mites to your home party, and they aren't the best guests. Use a dehumidifier if needed, like your home's personal climate control.

- **Avoid Smoking Indoors:** Just like you wouldn't puff away in your car, keep your home smoke-free. Smoking indoors is like giving your indoor air a nicotine kick, and we're not fans of that. Keep it fresh and clean!

- **Pets and Allergens:** If you have furry friends, they can carry allergens on their fur, like you're driving with the windows down. Groom them regularly and vacuum your home like a champion pit crew to reduce allergens. Your home, your rules!

- **Regular Cleaning:** Regular cleaning is like giving your home a spa day. Dust, sweep, mop, and wash bedding, curtains, and rugs. It's like getting your home all dressed up for a grand occasion - your comfort.

## Safety Measures and Emergency Plans

Now, let's talk about safety. Your home needs a safety belt, too:

- **Emergency Contacts:** Keep a list of emergency contacts near your phone or on the fridge - your safety crew. Whether it's your healthcare provider or family members, it's like your home's emergency hotline.

- **Fire Safety:** Install smoke detectors and carbon monoxide detectors and check them regularly, just like tuning up your car. Have a fire escape plan and make sure everyone in your household knows it. Safety first, just like on the road.

- **Emergency Kit:** Create an emergency kit, your home's version of a toolbox. Include essentials like medications, a list of your medical conditions, a first-aid kit, and non-perishable food and water. It's like having a pit stop for unexpected bumps in the road.

- **Power Outages:** Consider a backup power source like a generator. It's like having a spare tire for your home, ensuring that essential medical equipment can still run during power outages. Power up, even when the lights are out!

By crafting a COPD-friendly home environment, improving indoor air quality, and having safety measures and emergency plans in place, you're turning your home into a heaven where you can breathe easily and live comfortably. Your home, like a trusted road trip buddy, should be a place of comfort, safety, and peace on your COPD journey. It's your very own pit stop for a breath of fresh air.

"Patients at every stage of COPD can learn to work with their limitations, rather than against them."

Chapter 10:

# Monitoring Your COPD – Keeping Your Engine in Check

In this chapter we'll dive into the world of monitoring your COPD. Think of it as giving your lungs the same care you'd give your beloved car. So buckle up, and let's hit the road to learn about keeping a symptom diary, the importance of check-ups, and using peak flow meters or spirometers to keep your lung health in tip-top shape.

## Keeping a Symptom Diary

Consider a symptom diary for your car's maintenance log, but for your lungs. Here's how to create one:

- **Record Your Symptoms:** This is like noting down your car's performance issues but with a COPD twist. Jot down any changes in your breathing, cough, or mucus production. Include details like when they occur, how long they last, and their intensity. It's like sharing your car's hiccups with your mechanic but, in this case, with your healthcare provider.

- **Identify Triggers:** Just as your car might act up on bumpy roads, COPD symptoms can worsen due to triggers like smoke, allergens, or infections. Note when you're exposed to these triggers and how they affect you. It's like figuring out the potholes on your journey and avoiding them, COPD-style.

- **Track Medications:** Your symptom diary is like the car's record of when it had its last oil change. Keep a list of your medications, dosages, and when you take them. This ensures you're on top of your treatment plan, keeping your engine purring smoothly.

## Regular Check-Ups with Your Healthcare Provider

Just like routine car inspections keep potential issues at bay, regular check-ups benefit your COPD management:

- **Scheduled Appointments:** Think of these appointments as your car's oil change; don't skip them! Regular check-ups help assess your lung health and the effectiveness of your treatment. It's like having a professional mechanic inspect your engine regularly.

- **Review Your Symptom Diary:** Share your symptom diary with your healthcare provider. They can use it to understand how your COPD is progressing and make necessary adjustments to your treatment plan. It's like handing over your car's maintenance log to your trusted mechanic.

- **Update Your Action Plan:** If you have an action plan for managing exacerbations, review and update it with your healthcare provider as needed. Ensure it's like a well-maintained toolbox ready for any unexpected issues on the road. You wouldn't leave home without your car's toolbox, right?

## How to Use a Peak Flow Meter or Spirometer

Peak flow meters and spirometers are like diagnostic tools for your car; they help you measure lung function. Here's how to use them to monitor your COPD:

- **Peak Flow Meter:** Think of it as a fuel gauge for your lungs. To use it, follow these steps:
  a. Stand up straight and take a deep breath.
  b. Place the mouthpiece of the peak flow meter in your mouth and create a good seal around it.
  c. Blow out as hard and fast as you can into the meter. The meter will provide a reading of your peak flow.

It's like checking your car's fuel gauge to see if you have enough energy for the day.

- **Spirometer:** This tool measures how well you can inhale and exhale. To use it, follow these steps:
  a. Sit up straight and create a good seal around the spirometer's mouthpiece.
  b. Inhale as deeply as possible.
  c. Exhale forcefully into the spirometer as long as you can.
  d. The spirometer will provide readings of your lung function, including forced vital capacity (FVC) and forced expiratory volume in one second (FEV1).
  It's like getting a diagnostic scan of your car's engine during regular inspections.

Regularly monitoring your COPD is like routine car maintenance – it keeps your "engine" running smoothly. With a symptom diary, regular check-ups, and the use of peak flow meters or spirometers, you can stay on top of your COPD management. Just like a car needs an oil change and a check-up, your lungs need some care too. So, be diligent, stay on track, and keep your COPD under control with a smile!

"COPD affects much more than just your lungs. It affects your soul. But you can conquer it."

Chapter 11:

# Emotional Well-being – Nurturing Your Spirit

Let's talk about the emotional pit stop on your COPD journey. Just like a road trip, living with COPD comes with its fair share of twists and turns, and sometimes, it can feel like you've hit a few potholes along the way. In this chapter, we'll explore the importance of nurturing your emotional well-being, sharing experiences from both sides of the pond.

## Coping with Anxiety and Depression

Emotions are like the dashboard lights of your car, but instead of telling you when the engine's overheating, they signal feelings like anxiety and depression. So, how do we manage these emotional speed bumps?

- **Acknowledge Your Feelings:** First and foremost, it's essential to recognize and accept your emotions. It's okay to feel anxious, sad, or frustrated sometimes. Think of it like reading the dashboard of your emotional car; those emotions are the warning lights, and it's time to take action.

- **Communication is Key:** Talk to your healthcare provider about your emotional well-being. They're like the expert mechanics who can fix your engine when it's acting up. Sharing your struggles can lead to solutions and a smoother ride ahead.

- **Practice Mindfulness:** Techniques such as deep breathing and meditation are your pit stops for calming your mind. They help you stay in the present moment and manage anxious thoughts. It's like taking a scenic detour to enjoy the journey, rather than stressing about the destination.

- **Engage in Relaxation Techniques:** Relaxation methods, such as yoga and progressive muscle relaxation, are like a spa day for your soul. They help you manage stress and find inner peace. It's like fine-tuning your engine, ensuring it runs smoothly even when the road is rough.

## Support Groups and Mental Health Resources

Imagine support groups as the companions you meet at a rest stop during your road trip. They're there to offer guidance and a listening ear. How can they be valuable for your emotional well-being?

- **Support Groups:** COPD support groups are like those travelers who understand the road you're on. They provide a space for sharing experiences, tips, and encouragement, whether you're driving on the left side of the road in the UK or the right side in the USA.

- **Professional Help:** Mental health professionals, such as counselors or therapists, are your navigators. They offer guidance and strategies to manage anxiety and depression, ensuring a smoother journey, whether you're navigating London's winding streets or cruising through LA's boulevards.

- **Mental Health Resources:** Online resources and books about managing anxiety and depression are like your trusty GPS, helping you navigate your emotional journey. They provide insights and practical tips, no matter which side of the Atlantic you call home.

## Stay Engaged and Socialize

Your social life is like the playlist in your car, making the journey enjoyable. Here's how staying engaged and socializing can brighten your emotional well-being:

- **Stay Connected:** Just as you wouldn't drive alone for long distances, staying connected with family and friends is essential. Share your feelings and experiences with loved ones, whether you're catching up over a cuppa in the UK or sipping iced tea in the USA.

- **Engage in Hobbies:** Hobbies and interests are like scenic routes on your journey. They add enjoyment and purpose to your life, reducing feelings of isolation. Whether you're enjoying a pint at the local pub or savoring BBQ ribs, find the activities that bring you joy.

- **Volunteer or Join Clubs:** Volunteering or joining clubs and groups that match your interests is like making friends at a roadside café. It helps you meet new people, share experiences, and stay engaged.

- **Online Communities:** Online forums and social media groups dedicated to COPD provide a virtual road where you can connect with others. Even from the comfort of your home, it's like having a digital road trip, meeting new people without leaving your living room.

By acknowledging your feelings, seeking support from professionals and support groups, and staying engaged and socializing, you can nurture your emotional well-being on your COPD journey. Just like travelers on both sides of the pond, you can find comfort and companionship on the road, making the ride smoother and more enjoyable, regardless of the challenges you may face.

"By understanding both the physical and emotional aspects of COPD, you can learn to work with your problems rather than against them."

Chapter 12:

# Nutrition and COPD – Fueling Your Body

In this chapter we'll feast our eyes on the vital role of nutrition in managing COPD. Just as a plane needs the right fuel to soar through the skies, your body needs the right nutrients to navigate the COPD journey effectively. So, buckle up and join us for a culinary adventure as we explore nutrition's critical role in managing COPD.

## Understanding the Connection

Consider your body as a high-powered spaceship, and the food you eat as the rocket fuel propelling it. For those with COPD, nutrition isn't just about filling your belly; it's about supporting your lung health. Let's blast off into what you need to know:

- **The Energy Equation:** Your body, especially with COPD, works like a spaceship gearing up for an interstellar voyage. It needs extra energy to breathe efficiently. Like a spacecraft using more fuel to break through Earth's atmosphere, you require the right number of calories.
- **Maintaining Muscle Strength:** Think of your muscles as the space shuttle's engines. Just as they need fuel to fire up, your muscles, including those used for breathing, need proper nutrition to stay strong and ready for liftoff.
- **Reducing Inflammation:** COPD can be like a meteor shower causing chaos in your airways. Anti-inflammatory foods can act as your protective shields, helping to minimize the interstellar dust and debris.

## Dietary Guidelines for COPD

Navigating the galaxy of dietary guidelines can be as complex as calculating a space shuttle's trajectory. Here's how to set your course:

- **Balanced Diet:** Your dietary ship should be a sleek, well-rounded star cruiser, packed with an assortment of nutrient-rich foods. Think of your plate as the control panel: it should include fruits, vegetables, lean proteins, whole grains, and healthy fats to ensure a safe voyage.

- **Calorie Intake:** Whether you're launching from Earth or exploring the far reaches of the galaxy, the right amount of rocket fuel is crucial. If you're underweight, you may need more fuel to keep your engine running, while if you're carrying extra cargo, reducing your calorie consumption can lighten the load.

- **Protein:** Protein is your spaceship's building material. It's like the sturdy alloys that hold your craft together. Aim for lean proteins like poultry, fish, beans, and low-fat dairy to repair and build muscle, just as you'd ensure your ship's structure is solid for space travel.

- **Fiber:** Fiber-rich foods act as your spaceship's navigation system, keeping your journey smooth and your digestive system free of cosmic debris. A diet rich in whole grains, fruits, and vegetables ensures that your systems are in tip-top shape.

- **Omega-3 Fatty Acids:** Omega-3-rich foods are your space-age engines, allowing you to glide through the galaxy with ease. They help reduce inflammation and improve lung function, ensuring your journey is smooth and symptom-free.

## Staying Hydrated

Imagine proper hydration as your spaceship's coolant system, preventing overheating as you traverse the stars. Why is staying hydrated crucial for people with COPD?

- **Mucus Production:** Staying hydrated helps maintain the right viscosity of mucus in your airways. This prevents blockages and keeps your cosmic air passages clear, reducing coughing and breathlessness.

- **Medication Absorption:** Some COPD medications work like spacecraft upgrades, improving your systems and making your voyage more manageable. Proper hydration helps these medications do their job effectively.

- **Overall Well-being:** Staying hydrated is essential for your general health. It helps maintain energy levels, repair cosmic wear and tear, and keeps you running efficiently.

## Dietary Modifications for Specific Symptoms

Just as you'd adjust your spaceship's settings for different celestial environments, you can modify your diet to address specific COPD symptoms:

- **Bloating and Gas:** If you experience excessive bloating and gas, consider smaller, more frequent "meal orbits." Avoid cosmic foods that cause gas, and keep carbonated beverages off your menu.
- **Difficulty Swallowing:** Swallowing challenges are like navigating asteroid fields. Stick to softer, mashed, or pureed foods, and chew thoroughly. You don't want to choke on space debris!
- **Weight Management:** Your spaceship's cargo load is a critical factor for your journey. Work with a dietary navigator to create a plan that helps you reach and maintain a healthy, well-balanced cosmic weight.

## Nutrition as Your Cosmic Copilot

Just as a wise copilot helps you navigate through the cosmos, nutrition can be your partner in managing COPD. By understanding the importance of nutrition, following dietary guidelines, staying well-hydrated, and making dietary adjustments when necessary, you can ensure that your spaceship is fueled for a seamless journey with COPD. So, set your course, keep your engines firing, and explore the universe of better lung health with the right dietary choices.

"Millions of people worldwide have COPD but are currently undiagnosed."

Chapter 13:

# Effective Communication – The Road to Understanding

Just as you wouldn't attempt a cross-country road trip without a map and some good tunes, navigating your path with COPD requires clear and open communication. So, let's get talking!

## Discussing Your Condition with Family and Friends

Picture your loved ones as the trusted co-pilots in your life's adventure. Just like you'd keep them in the loop during a road trip, sharing your COPD experience with family and friends is vital:

- **Open and Honest Dialogue:** Effective communication begins with open and honest dialogue. Share your feelings, challenges, and fears with your loved ones. Think of it as gathering your fellow travelers for a pre-road-trip pow-wow.
- **Education:** Educate your family and friends about COPD. Help them understand the condition, its symptoms, and the impact it has on your daily life. Knowledge is like the ultimate GPS, guiding them in supporting you effectively.
- **Set Realistic Expectations:** Communication isn't just about sharing; it's also about setting realistic expectations. Let your loved ones know about your limitations and when you might need a little extra support. It's like planning pit stops on a long car journey.
- **Expressing Gratitude:** Don't forget to express gratitude for their support. Acknowledging their efforts is like sharing your snacks with your fellow travelers – it keeps the journey enjoyable.

## Effective Communication with Healthcare Professionals

Your healthcare provider is your ultimate GPS in your COPD journey, guiding you to the best destinations. Effective communication with them is key:

- **Prepare for Appointments:** Just as you'd prepare for a road trip with a checklist, before visiting your healthcare provider, make a list of questions, concerns, and symptoms. It's like getting your checklist ready for a pit stop.

- **Be Honest and Transparent:** Be honest and transparent about your COPD symptoms, lifestyle, and medication adherence. Your healthcare provider can only help if they have all the details, just like your mechanic fixing your car.
- **Seek Clarification:** If you don't understand something your healthcare provider says, don't hesitate to seek clarification. Asking questions is like stopping at a gas station to ask for directions when you're unsure of the route.
- **Collaborate on Treatment Plans:** Your healthcare provider is like your co-pilot on this journey. Collaborate on your treatment plan, and make sure you both agree on the best approach for managing your COPD. Think of it as discussing the route and pit stops with your co-pilot on a road trip.

## Advance Care Planning and End-of-Life Decisions

Advance care planning is like choosing the scenic route for the rest of your journey – it's a bit challenging, but oh so necessary:

- **Advance Directives:** Create advance directives, including a living will and durable power of attorney for healthcare. Think of these documents as your last will and testament for your journey, ensuring your wishes are respected.
- **Discuss End-of-Life Wishes:** Have open and honest conversations with your family and healthcare provider about your end-of-life wishes. It's like discussing your dream travel destinations – talk about your preferences for medical care and interventions.
- **Review and Update:** Just as you'd revise your travel itinerary for unexpected detours, regularly review and update your advance care planning documents. Life's journey may take unexpected turns, and it's essential to ensure your documents reflect your current wishes.
- **Seek Support:** Coping with advance care planning can be emotionally challenging. Seek support from healthcare professionals, social workers, or support groups to help navigate this part of your journey. Think of it as getting travel advice from a

seasoned traveler – sometimes, you need a pro to guide you through the tricky bits.

Effective communication is your trusty road map, whether you're sharing your COPD experience with loved ones, talking to healthcare professionals, or addressing advance care planning and end-of-life decisions. As you navigate this journey, remember, a little humor, a lot of patience, and clear communication can make all the difference. So, let's keep those conversations going and ensure you're heard loud and clear on this road with COPD.

"The only way to truly understand COPD is to live it."

Chapter 14:

# Traveling with COPD – Navigating the Road and Skies

Just like you'd gear up for a road trip with your trusty map and favorite snacks, preparing for trips and vacations with COPD requires some careful planning. It's all about ensuring you have your medications, documents, and the right attitude to deal with air travel and changing altitudes. So, fasten your seatbelts, and let's embark on this journey!

## Preparing for Trips and Vacations

Think of your travel preparations as the ultimate road trip checklist – meticulous planning is the key to a successful adventure. Here's how to ensure your travels go off without a hitch:

- **Consult Your Healthcare Provider:** Just as you'd inspect your car before a long journey, pay your doctor a visit before you hit the road. Discuss your travel plans, destination, and any specific concerns you may have. It's like getting your car inspected to avoid breakdowns in the middle of nowhere.
- **Pack Medications and Supplies:** Remember to pack your COPD medications, inhalers, and any necessary medical supplies. Ensure you have more than enough to last the duration of your trip. Think of it as packing a trusty first-aid kit for any unexpected emergencies.
- **Create an Emergency Plan:** Your trip needs an emergency plan, just like a road trip requires a breakdown plan. Know where the nearest medical facilities are, and have a list of emergency contacts. It's like having a roadmap to your nearest pit stop.
- **Know Your Limitations:** Recognize your energy levels and know when to take breaks. Plan your activities accordingly, ensuring you don't overexert yourself. It's akin to scheduling rest stops during a long drive to recharge.

## Carrying Necessary Medications and Documents

As you gear up for your adventure, make sure you've got all the right documents and medications in your arsenal. It's like carrying your ID and vehicle registration for a road trip – essential and non-negotiable:

- **Medication List:** Create a detailed list of your medications, including names, dosages, and schedules. Keep a copy in your wallet or bag in case of an emergency. Think of it as an essential document in your car's glove compartment.
- **Prescription Copies:** Always carry copies of your prescriptions, especially for controlled medications. They can be vital when traveling or in case your medications are lost or stolen. It's like having proof of insurance for your car.
- **Medical ID Card:** Consider getting a medical ID card or bracelet that specifies your condition. This can be crucial in case of a medical emergency where you're unable to communicate. It's like your car's identification number for easy recognition.
- **Travel Insurance:** Invest in travel insurance, just like you'd opt for comprehensive car insurance. It provides coverage in case of unexpected events like trip cancellations, medical emergencies, or lost baggage. It's your safety net for unforeseen incidents.

## Coping with Air Travel and Changing Altitudes

Air travel can be a breeze, but for those with COPD, it requires some special considerations. Here's how to manage air travel effectively:

- **Notify the Airline:** When booking your flight, let the airline know about your condition. This allows them to make necessary arrangements and provide assistance as needed. It's like requesting special services for your car before a long journey.
- **Carry Medications in Your Carry-On:** Just as you'd carry essential items in your handbag or backpack, ensure your COPD medications are in your carry-on bag. This ensures you have access to them during the flight, just like your car's essentials are in the glove compartment.
- **Stay Hydrated:** Like maintaining optimal engine temperature in a car, staying hydrated is crucial during air travel. Drink water regularly to prevent dehydration – consider it the equivalent of keeping your car's engine temperature from overheating.

- **Exercise While Seated:** Prevent stiffness and discomfort during the flight by performing seated exercises. Ankle circles, knee lifts, and shoulder rolls can keep your blood circulating. It's like checking your car's tire pressure during a long drive to ensure smooth performance.
- **Consult Your Doctor for Long Flights:** If you're taking a long-haul flight, consult your doctor. They may recommend specific measures, such as adjusting your medication schedule or using supplemental oxygen during the flight. Think of it as having your car inspected before a cross-country road trip.

Traveling with COPD is all about planning and preparation. With the right mindset, necessary medications and documents, and a solid plan for air travel, you can explore new horizons and enjoy your adventures while effectively managing your condition. So, embrace the wanderlust, and let your COPD journey be as memorable as the travel itself.

"Life is not measured by the number of breaths we take, but by the moments that take our breath away"

Chapter 15:

# Charting New Horizons – Your Journey of Resilience

Congratulations, dear reader! You've journeyed through the pages of this book, delving into the world of COPD, learning about its challenges, and discovering how to navigate life's twists and turns with this condition. But always remember, it's your happiness that matters most.

## 1. Your Life Is Like a Beautiful Mosaic

Think of your life as a grand masterpiece, like a vibrant mosaic where each piece represents a unique experience, be it a challenge or a triumph. The beauty of a mosaic lies in the sum of its parts, the colors, the shapes, and the story it tells. Your life is just like that – every moment, every challenge you've overcome, and every joy you've felt are the pieces that come together to create a masterpiece.

COPD might be one piece in your mosaic, but it's not the only piece. It's a part of your story, but it doesn't define the whole narrative. Embrace the colorful pieces of your life – your family, your friends, your hobbies, your passions – and keep adding more. Each day is a chance to create new, vibrant tiles in your mosaic.

## 2. The Small Victories Matter Most

When you live with COPD, it's easy to focus on the big battles, but don't underestimate the small victories. Celebrate those everyday moments – the deep breath you manage to take, the laughter shared with a friend, the sunny days that lift your spirits. These small wins are the building blocks of a joyful life.

Appreciate the simple pleasures, like the smell of freshly baked bread, the feel of a warm, cozy blanket, or the sound of your favorite song. Happiness often resides in these small, ordinary moments, so keep them close to your heart. And remember, when you add up all these small victories, they create a beautiful life worth living.

### 3. Your Story Inspires Others

Your journey with COPD is unique, and it's a story that can inspire others. Your experiences, your strength, and your resilience can motivate those around you. You may not even realize the impact your story has on the people you meet.

Think about how you've overcome the challenges and how you've learned to embrace life with a smile. Share your story, not as a tale of struggle but as a narrative of triumph. The wisdom you've gained is invaluable, and it can light the path for others who are on a similar journey.

## 4. Learn, Adapt, and Thrive

Throughout this book, you've learned about COPD, its management, and the strategies to enhance your well-being. Now, take that knowledge and continue adapting, evolving, and thriving.

Life is an ever-changing landscape, and as you navigate through it, you'll discover new ways to overcome obstacles. Use your wisdom and resourcefulness to your advantage. You're not just a passenger on this journey; you're the driver, and you have the power to steer in the direction of happiness.

## 5. Love, Laughter, and Adventure Await

Always remember that love, laughter, and adventure are always within reach. Whether it's the love of family and friends, the joy of shared laughter, or the thrill of new experiences, there's a world full of wonderful moments waiting for you.

Travel to new places, try out new hobbies, and savor new cuisines. Bask in the joy of celebrations, milestones, and cherished traditions. Let your life be a vibrant tapestry of experiences and emotions. Fill it with the love of your dear ones, the warmth of hugs, and the sound of hearty laughter.

## 6. Stay Curious and Keep Dreaming

Embrace your curiosity. Keep dreaming. The world is an intriguing place with countless things to explore and discover. Be open to new interests, hobbies, and passions. The excitement of learning and the thrill of discovery can add a thrilling layer to your journey.

Remember, age is just a number, and dreams have no expiration date. Let your curiosity lead you down new paths. Your dreams, both big and small, are the stars that guide your adventure. Whether it's learning a new language, taking up painting, or traveling to a dream destination, your desires are the compass for your journey.

## 7. Every Sunrise Is a New Beginning

Each day, when you wake up to a new sunrise, it's a fresh start, a new beginning. Leave yesterday's worries behind and step into the new day with optimism. Consider it a blank canvas waiting for the strokes of your choices and actions.

No matter what's happened in the past, every sunrise is a reminder that you have the chance to create a better today. Focus on the positive, set goals, and look forward to the surprises life has in store. As the day unfolds, relish in the beauty of the present moment, for it's the gift you've been given.

## 8. Gratitude Is Your Travel Companion

Gratitude is the map that leads you to joy. Cultivate this beautiful quality, for it can turn the ordinary into the extraordinary. Every day, take a moment to reflect on the things you're grateful for. Your family, your friends, the small victories, and even the challenges that have made you stronger.

Gratitude can transform your perspective, reminding you of the abundance in your life. It's a magnifying glass that amplifies the beauty around you. Keep it close as you journey forward, and it will fill your life with contentment and joy.

## 9. You Are Not Alone on This Journey

Remember, you are not alone on this journey. Your loved ones, your healthcare providers, and countless others are here to support you. They're your co-pilots, your fellow adventurers, and your friends along the way.

Share your thoughts, your fears, and your dreams with them. Lean on them when you need assistance or simply a listening ear. Just as you've learned to communicate effectively in the previous chapter, continue reaching out and fostering connections. You're part of a grand community, and together, you can create a vibrant, supportive network.

## 10. The Best Is Yet to Come

Believe in the magic of the unknown. Every corner turned, every path chosen, and every journey embarked upon holds the promise of something wonderful. The best is yet to come, and it's waiting for you.

So, as we conclude this book, remember, your journey with COPD is a unique, colorful adventure. The road ahead is filled with reasons to embrace life – from the small victories to the inspiring stories you'll collect along the way. Your life is a beautiful mosaic, and each piece, no matter how big or small, contributes to the masterpiece that is uniquely yours.

As you venture forward, use the knowledge you've acquired, the resilience you've nurtured, and the optimism you've embraced to create a life that's rich, fulfilling, and filled with love, laughter, and adventure. With each sunrise, cherish the new beginning it brings. Stay curious, keep dreaming, and let gratitude be your constant companion. You are not alone on this journey – countless hands are extended, ready to offer support and share in your joy.

Finally, remember that the best is yet to come. Your journey with COPD is not an end but a beginning, and the adventures ahead are worth every step. Embrace life with open arms and an open heart, for your story is a beautiful tale waiting to be written. You are the author, and your journey is the adventure of a lifetime.

www.ingramcontent.com/pod-product-compliance
Lightning Source LLC
Chambersburg PA
CBHW080855260726
48660CB00009B/3315